Easy Juicing Recipes

Athletes Energy Drink To Improve Your Energy And Increase Your Performance

Fabian Mendez

Introduction

I want to thank you and congratulate you for downloading the book, *"Easy Juicing Recipes - Athletes Energy Drink To Improve Your Energy And Increase Your Performance."*

Swimmers, runners, and cyclists use juice to gain the energy they need to compete against their rivals while increasing their endurance. Juices will not necessarily make you faster, but they will help you maintain peak performance for longer.

Sports energy drinks are beverages specially formulated to help you as an athlete rehydrate during or after a performance. Adequate hydration decreases chances of cramping, as cramping hampers performance depending on the heat and the duration.

However, what we do know about commercial sports drinks is that they are full of empty carbs in the form of sugar. While this is instant energy for an athlete, most of these drinks have zero nutrients and often leave you craving for more.

To avoid this and instead drink juices that energize you and increase your performance, you need to make your own juices from fruits and other ingredients.

In this guide, we will be discussing the best juice recipes you can use to develop a lean and mean body that allows you to perform at your best while avoiding inflammation.

Thanks again for downloading this book, I hope you enjoy it!

Table of Contents

Chapter 1: What Should Be In A Sports Drink?

The right sports energy drink should be rich in carbohydrates, which is obviously the most efficient source of energy. It should also contain electrolytes that are lost along with body fluid as we sweat. Electrolytes are positive ions in our bodies that are charged for electrical conduction. They are from minerals like sodium, magnesium, calcium, and potassium. The main reason electrolytes are important in an athlete's body is that they are responsible for maintaining the right PH levels. Correct PH levels create electrical impulse balance that promotes muscle cell functions during exercise.

Normally, sweat rates will differ. You may be the athlete who loses 1 kg of water heavily concentrated with high levels of sodium or one who loses 3kgs of water but with very little potassium or sodium. What matters is replacement of these electrolytes to promote rehydration for the purposes of delaying the onset of fatigue during exercise.

Types Of Sport Drinks

Sports drinks vary depending on the levels of carbohydrates, electrolytes, and fluid in them. Nevertheless, there are three kinds of sports drinks: **hypotonic, hypertonic**, and **isotonic** sports drink.

Hypotonic drinks contain a lower concentration of salt and sugar than our bodies. They quickly replace the fluid you may have lost through sweating. This type of drink is suitable for athletes who need fluid without a boost of their carbohydrate levels.

Hypertonic drinks contain a higher concentration of sugar and salt than what is in our bodies. This kind of drink works best when consumed after a work out to supplement the daily carbohydrate intake and top-up glycogen stores in the muscles. You can also use it during a long distance event to meet the high-energy demands alongside an isotonic energy drink to replace lost fluid.

Isotonic drinks have the same levels of salt and sugar as our body. The work of these drinks is to replace the fluids we lose through sweating and to boost our carbohydrate levels. This drink is most suitable for middle and long distance runners.

Chapter 2: Natural Sports Drinks

The sports drink market has many confusing and often conflicting brands; as such, it is hard to tell which ones are the best for you as an athlete. Obviously, pure clean water is the best.

Our bodies are 70% water and we lose a lot of it when we work out. It is therefore a rule of thumb that we drink at least 8 glasses of water on a normal day and more when in the field. Water helps transport oxygen and glucose throughout the body, helps maintain flexibility, and strengthens your muscles while at the same time lubricating your joints.

Failure to drink enough water could cause headaches and decreases in energy, which are all warning signs of dehydration. The problem is that after a while, plain water can get boring and it does not contain high levels of the electrolytes you lose as you exercise; hence the need to make your own natural energy drink.

Before stopping by the store to buy Gatorade on your way to the game, try making your own natural version of an energy drink: it is a lot healthier, easier, and just as fast. Why should you try making your own rather than reach for your regular store energy drinks?

Apart from the carbohydrates and electrolytes, regular sports drinks contain additional ingredients like monopotassium phosphate, natural flavors, and unnecessary artificial dyes. Some caffeinated drinks may also contain banned substances such as ephedrine, which might end up costing you your career as an athlete. A natural sports drink is a simple way out of all this.

Going natural means replacing store-bought energy drinks with juice made from fruits and vegetables. Because of their ability to improve endurance and performance, a number of major players hold some plants in high regard.

Here, we are talking about **celery**, **cucumbers**, **coconut water**, and **watermelons**. Any natural drink you juice should have at least one of them. Let us learn why each of these vegetables is important.

Celery

First, celery hydrates the body and helps keep the colon walls hydrated too. This helps get rid of hemorrhoids, a common problem you are likely to face when you are dehydrated and your diet lacks enough fiber.

Celery is also rich in electrolytes, mainly sodium and potassium. These two electrolytes combine with other electrolyte minerals in your body to provide your body with the necessary salt-ion balance that penetrates the cells and hydrates them. These two electrolytes present in celery make it ideal as the most complete fluid replacement drink.

It is important to note that sodium from common table salt or sodium chloride will not be as helpful in hydrating you. Instead, it causes bloating that upsets the stomach since it does not break down efficiently. As a result, your body sends a trigger to dump what is in the stomach. Your body perceives this as some sort of gastro intestinal threat and shuts your legs, ending your performance.

In addition to the sodium and potassium, celery also contains secondary minerals that serve the purpose of increasing your endurance. The calcium and magnesium in celery allows your muscles to continue the electrical impulse without fail even after their depletion. The main cause of cramping during and after a competition is lack of enough calcium and magnesium that are always responsible for expansion and retraction of the muscles.

When lactic acid piles up in your body, it becomes the number one limiting factor to performance. Another remarkable importance of drinking celery juice is that because of its diuretic effect, which it gets from sodium and potassium, it helps flush out these acids.

Cucumber

Many benefits in celery parallel cucumber's thus making it a great source of endurance too. Cucumbers have a water content of 96% and the nutrients in the juice cause a cooling effect in the body. This is important since the heat you produce affects your endurance as an athlete. By drinking cucumber juice, you bring down your overall body temperature, which extends your performance.

Cucumbers are also a great source of magnesium and potassium. Cucumber also has a diuretic effect that will help get rid of excess fluid in the body. Further, since the juice is alkaline in nature, it naturally helps generate energy.

The other importance of cucumber juice is that it is a great source of silica, which is a building block for your body. Your ligaments, bones, muscles, and other connective tissues use silica as a major rebuilding and repair component. Cucumber is also rich in copper, primarily responsible for moving energy around the body.

In addition, because of the other minerals it has like molybdenum, sulfur, folate, vitamin A and vitamin C, cucumber makes it possible for your body to assimilate and boost endurance.

Coconut Water

Reasons why you should add coconut water to your hydration drink are many.

First, coconut water is the most pure form of water that does not need any further distilling probably because its purification started from the ground to 30-40ft high. It is practically impossible to find any other liquid on the planet that has gone through the purification level coconut water goes through. Its purity is also because of the hard coconut shell that protects it from external elements.

Secondly, coconut water is rich in potassium; potassium boosts endurance. This electrolyte (potassium) travels to every cells in your body and is responsible for every electrical impulse for nerve conduction, the contraction of your heart, as well as skeletal muscle contraction.

Coconut water also has sodium. Sodium works to regulate the fluid in your body. Because it prevents body dehydration, it also helps flush out toxins and excess fluids. 14 ounces of coconut water contains approximately 192 mg of sodium compared to the 52 mg in Gatorade.

Because of its alkaline nature, coconut water falls in the isotonic drink category. This alkalinity makes it possible to neutralize and flash out the lactic acid in the cells and the muscles during exercise. Coconut water also contains phosphorous, an electrolyte that transfers energy throughout your body. Coconut water also has the ability to regulate your body temperature, which promotes competing for a long time without overheating.

Watermelon

Just like celery, coconut water, and cucumber, watermelon contains more than 90% water alongside the five major electrolytes. To be exact, watermelon contains 92% water, which makes it a mild diuretic. It is also rich in antioxidants like beta-carotene and lycopene that help the body protect itself from attack from sunlight, bacteria, and fungi.

Free radicals, if unchecked, can wreak havoc on your good health. For instance, they can oxidize cholesterol thus allowing it to stick to your arterial wall consequently causing strokes and heart attacks. Increased inflammation in the body, which causes rheumatoid arthritis and osteoarthritis, can also be a result of the free radicals.

The Lycopene in watermelon neutralizes these free radicals before they can start a negative chain reaction in your body. This is important to you as an athlete since your bone and joint health need to be in check for your endurance and output.

Watermelon is also rich in L-citrulline. This nutrient has an intense therapeutic effect on your muscles. Further, it extends the production of nitric oxide because the l-Arginie is recycled, which is the pre-cursor to nitric oxide.

L-citrulline also protects the l-arginine production by neutralizing the amino acid L-Arginase in the blood that destroys it. Drinking watermelon juice will give the body a more direct pathway to utilize the nitric oxide, which will boost your performance for a much longer period.

If you race in long distance marathons, bike race, or participate in ultra-endurance events, watermelon juice will keep you hydrated and deliver the essential nutrients your muscles need to maintain peak performance.

Chapter 3: Juices vs. Smoothies

Many of us tend to use these names interchangeably but freshly extracted juices are not the same as smoothies. To make smoothies, you blend fresh fruits to produce a delicious drink. This is different from extracted juice because a smoothie contains all the fiber present in the fruit.

When you place the same fruit in a juice extractor, you will end up separating the juice from the fiber. This is beneficial because you will get more nutrients from the juice without overworking your system with all that fiber. It also takes less time for the body to absorb the nutrients and your digestive system requires less energy to do so as compared to when you take the whole fruit.

Do not forget that fiber should be part of your diet so that your digestive system functions. Therefore, juices should not replace your fiber diet; rather, let the juices be an addition to a high fiber diet so that you can benefit from both.

Although fruit juices have many of the benefits mentioned above, making them green by adding vegetables would be an added advantage. Greens have a high chlorophyll content that will help oxygenate your blood. They are also rich in calcium, magnesium, and iron which are essential for your endurance. Greens also have low sugar content hence least impact in terms of blood sugar spikes.

Chapter 4: Juicing Recipes for Athletes

When selecting a juicer, choose a model that has a good quality motor (preferably 750 watts or more), one that is easy to clean, and is efficient at extracting juices from fruits, vegetables, and other leafy greens.

If you do not have a juicer, you can still use a powerful high-speed blender to blend your ingredients, and then use a fine mesh sieve to separate the liquid from chunks of veggies and all the fibers. Alternatively, you can get a big drawstring bag where you put all the pulp in there and squeeze your juice out.

If you are looking for a pre-workout energy drink or one you will drink during or after your game, the following healthy juice recipes have you covered. Enjoy!

Watermelon Cucumber Juice

Yield: 4 cups

Ingredients

4 organic lemon cucumbers or 1 large cucumber

4 cups of organic watermelon

Instructions

Cut the watermelon in half and using a spoon, scoop out chunks of its flesh to fill 4 measuring cups.

Cut the cucumbers into pieces, and then juice the cucumbers then the watermelon.

Serve immediately as is or with some ice.

Before The Gym Energy Drink

Yield: 1 serving

This drink contains Rhodiola as one of its ingredients. Rhodiola improves endurance during exercise while the combination of fructose from the berries and glucose will provide both short-term and long-term energy release.

Ingredients

1 cup of frozen berries

1 scoop of whey protein

1 tablespoon of glucose

1g of Rhodiola extract

500ml of filtered water

Instructions

Juice the berries and pour the resultant juice into a glass. Add in the other ingredients, stir, and enjoy.

Natural Electrolyte Drink

Yield: 4 servings

This drink is a great way to rehydrate after exercise. Unlike other store-bought drinks, this one does not have tons of sugar.

Ingredients

¼ cup of pineapple juice

2 tablespoons of sweetener

1 teaspoon of calcium magnesium powder

1/4 teaspoon of sea salt

1 quart of coconut water

Instructions

Slightly warm your coconut water, and then add sea salt and calcium to the mix.

Add sweetener, juice, and then mix.

Refrigerate until when ready to drink.

Energy Drink

Yield: 1 serving

This drink is full of proteins and vitamins that will give you the long lasting energy boost you will need during your performance.

Ingredients

6 oz. of very light vanilla yoghurt

1 tablespoon of honey

¾ cups of light coconut milk

1 medium orange, peeled and cut

Instructions

Put the orange into your juicer and juice. Pour the juice into a glass, add the other ingredients, stir, and enjoy.

Beetroot Juice

Yield: 1 serving

The nitrate in the beets will open up you blood vessels, easing the transportation of oxygen to your muscles through the free flow of blood. Combining the beets with vegetables improves its taste and allows you to take a wider range of vitamins and nutrients.

Ingredients

1 clove of garlic

1 lemon with its rind

1 inch of ginger

2 kale leaves

3 carrots

1 fresh beet

Instructions

Juice all the ingredients and serve immediately to ensure you get the most nutrition.

High Protein Energy Drink

Yield: 2 servings

This drink is especially necessary if you are an athlete looking to build your muscles. In addition to lean meat, pineapples and kale make a great source of proteins alongside other healthy nutrients.

Ingredients

10 leaves of kale

1 big handful of parsley

1 inch-long knob of ginger

4 celery stalks

4 carrots

3 apples

1 pineapple

Instructions

Juice all the ingredients and enjoy.

Rocket Fuel Juice

Yield: 2 servings

This drink will help you feel less pain in your muscles even after a rigorous exercise.

Ingredients

½ organic lime with rind

1 organic cucumber with rind

1 large celery stalk

1 pound of Montmorency cherries, pitted

½ pound of fresh strawberries

1 green apple

Instructions

Place all the ingredients in a juicer and process. Serve immediately.

Tomato Juice

Yield: 1 serving

Lycopene is a compound found in tomatoes that not only enables faster tomato recovery, but also stabilizes blood sugar levels.

Ingredients

1 big handful of cilantro

1 tomato

1 organic lime with rind

1 organic lemon with rind

4 large carrots

Instructions

Place all the ingredients in a juicer and process to extract the juice. Serve immediately to enjoy the nutrients.

Athletes Juice

Yield: 1L

Ingredients

2-inch piece of ginger

8 kale leaves

1 large handful of parsley

3 celery stalks

4 carrots

3 apples

½ pineapple

Instructions

Peel the ginger and remove the rind from the pineapple.

Wash all the ingredients and process them in the juicer.

Serve and enjoy.

Race-day Juice

Yield: 1 serving

Ingredients

5 strawberries

½ lemon, pulped

2 beets, cut into quarters

Instructions

Put all your ingredients in a juice extractor and process until ready. Serve.

Immune Booster

Yield: 1 serving

Ingredients

10 grapes

1 orange, cut into small pieces

1 cucumber

3 kale leaves

Instructions

Put all ingredients in a juice extractor and process. Serve.

Post-race Recovery Juice

Yield: 1 serving

Ingredients

1 inch ginger root

1 cup of blueberries

2 cups of tart cherries, seeded.

Instructions

Put all ingredients in a juice extractor and process. Serve.

Orange and Broccoli Juice

Yield: 1 serving

Kiwifruit, orange, and broccoli are excellent sources of vitamin C necessary for the production of collagen. Collagen is the protein we need to maintain healthy skin, bones, and cartilage. This drink also provides iron, potassium, and vitamin A.

Ingredients

1 kiwifruit, peeled and chopped

1 cup (125g) of broccoli, chopped

1 large orange, peeled, seeded and chopped

Instructions

Process all the ingredients in a juicer and serve.

Pear and Peach Juice

Yield: 1 serving

These fruits have a low glycemic index giving a slow release of energy. It is therefore a good drink to have an hour before your workout or performance.

Ingredients

Filtered or spring water to taste

2 apricots, pitted and chopped

1 peach, unpeeled, pitted, and chopped

1 peer unpeeled, cored and chopped

Instructions

Process all the fruits in a juicer. Thin with a small amount of water if need be and enjoy.

Cucumber and Parsley Juice

Yield: 1 serving

Orange supplies vitamin C that helps your body utilize the iron in parsley. On the other hand, cucumber has a cooling effect and therefore useful after an event or workout.

Spirulina is a "super food" high in many nutrients.

Ingredients

½ teaspoon of Spirulina powder

1 small cucumber

2 cups packed parsley spring with stems

1 large orange, peeled, seeded and chopped.

Instructions

Process the parsley, orange, and cucumber in a juicer and pour into a glass.

Stir in the Spirulina powder and serve.

Plum and Berry Juice

Yield: 1 serving

Go for the red-fleshed plum variety; they are higher in nutrients than the yellow-fleshed one. Plums are also rich in potassium electrolyte alongside vitamins A, C, and E. The berries provide vitamin C and bioflavonoids that strengthen arteries and veins.

Ingredients

3 large red-fleshed plums, pitted and chopped

1 cup (125g) of frozen strawberries, thawed

1 cup (125g) blackberries, frozen and thawed

Instructions

Process all the ingredients in a juicer and serve immediately.

Cantaloupe Juice

Yield: 1 serving

The vitamin C in pineapple and guava encourage the production of collagen, a protein that fosters healthy bones and cartilage. Cantaloupe and pineapple have a high water content that is good for rehydration. Pineapple is also rich in an enzyme called bromelain, which is an anti-inflammatory that promotes the repair of damaged tissues caused by sporting activities.

Ingredients

1 guava, unpeeled and cut into wedges

¼ pineapple, peeled, cored, and chopped

¼ cantaloupe, peeled, seeded and chopped

Instructions

Process all the ingredients in a juicer and serve.

Pineapple Juice

Yield: 2 serving

Fennel is a female reproductive tonic that could be very useful to menstrual problems in female athletes. This juice is not only refreshing; it is also rich in antioxidants, vitamins, and enzymes.

Ingredients

¼ fennel bulb, trimmed, cored, and chopped

1 lime, peeled, seeded, and chopped

¼ papaya, peeled, seeded, and chopped

½ pineapple, peeled, cored, and chopped

Instructions

Put all ingredients in a juicer and process; serve.

Melon and Grape Juice

Yield: 1 serving

Melons and lychees have a cooling effect on your body. This juice is therefore great to have after a workout. Grapes replenish energy first because they have a high glycemic index.

Ingredients

6 lychees, peeled and seeded

1 cup (125g) of grapes

½ small honeydew melon, peeled, seeded and chopped

Instructions

Process all the ingredients in a juicer.

Serve and enjoy.

Carrot and Ginger Juice

Yield: 1 serving

Ginger helps to stimulate circulation and aids in digestion. Carrot and orange contain the important antioxidants vitamins A and C. Ginseng gives a natural energy boost.

Ingredients

½ inch piece of fresh ginger

1 large orange, peeled, seeded and chopped

1 large carrot, chopped

½ cup (125ml) boiling water

1 ginseng tea bag

Instructions

Steep the ginseng tea bag in a cup of boiling water for 10 minutes then remove.

Refrigerate the tea for about 20 minutes.

Process the ginger, orange, and carrot in a juicer and pour into a cup.

Pour in the tea and stir to combine.

Serve and enjoy.

Papaya and Mango Juice

Yield: 1 serving

Because papaya and mango have a high glycemic index, this juice makes a great drink after an exercise or a performance; it quickly restores your lost energy.

Ingredients

1 mango, peeled, cut from pit and chopped

¼ papaya, peeled, seeded and chopped

1 ruby grapefruit, peeled, seeded, and chopped

Instructions

Process all the ingredients in a juicer and then serve.

Tomato and Cabbage Juice

Yield: 1 serving

Tomatoes, celery, and cabbage contain potassium and sodium electrolytes that are important for balancing the electrolytes in your body. Celery also has anti-inflammatory properties. This drink is therefore a good one to have after a workout.

Ingredients

2 celery stalks

1 cup (30g) of packed parsley springs with stems

1 1/3 cups (125 g) cabbage, chopped

1 ripe tomato, cut into wedges

Instructions

Process all the ingredients in a juicer and serve.

Chapter 5: Juice Recipes To Fight Inflammation

Inflammation of the muscles or in the body is never a good thing for athletes. These juice recipes will help you fight inflammation:

Green Juice

Yield: 1 serving

If you frequently feel low on energy, you may be anemic. The greens in this juice are a great source of iron. In addition, the ginger and lemon ensure maximum absorption and increase the speed of inflammation recovery.

Ingredients

1-inch ginger root

½ lemon

1 cucumber

A punch of parsley

2 green apples

8 leaves of kale

Instructions

Juice all the ingredients in your juicer, serve, and enjoy.

Green Pineapple Juice

Yield: 1 serving

The pineapple and ginger are effective anti-inflammatory foods that will help reduce inflammation and joint aches.

Ingredients

1-inch fresh ginger root

A few sprigs mint leaves

A big handful spinach

6 ribs of celery

1 cup of pineapple chunks

Instructions

Put all the ingredients in a juicer and process until ready. Serve and enjoy.

Ginger Beet Juice

Yield: 1 serving

If you routinely workout, then beetroot juice is a drink you should also routinely drink. Drinking it before your workout improves your stamina and endurance. Drinking it after helps reduce inflammation.

Ingredients

1-inch ginger root

1 small lemon

5 beetroots

Instructions

Juice all the ingredients and enjoy.

Conclusion

Thank you again for downloading this book!

Make an effort of making your own energy drinks, as you will know the exact ingredients in them, and you will be consuming fresh nutritious ingredients full of the natural vitamins and minerals your body needs to operate at peak performance.

Finally, if you enjoyed this book, would you be kind enough to leave a review for this book on Amazon?

Click here to leave a review for this book on Amazon!

If you have received value from this ebook I recommended to read my other ebook you can find it here

https://www.amazon.com/dp/B06Y4C2TDB

Thank you and good luck!

www.ingramcontent.com/pod-product-compliance
Lightning Source LLC
Chambersburg PA
CBHW071141280526
45787CB00003B/1358